Unlocking Alzheimer's Secrets

Decoding the Role of RNA in Neurodegeneration

By

Fletcher Paul

Table of contents

Chapter 1: Introduction

Alzheimer's disease stands as a formidable global health challenge, affecting approximately 55 million people worldwide. As we delve into understanding the intricacies of this devastating condition, it becomes paramount to explore its far-reaching impact on individuals, families, and societies at large.

The Global Impact of Alzheimer's Disease

Alzheimer's disease transcends geographical boundaries, leaving an indelible mark on diverse communities worldwide. Its prevalence has surged over the years, demanding attention due to the sheer magnitude of its impact on public health. Families grapple with the emotional and financial burdens associated with caring for loved ones affected by the disease. Moreover, healthcare systems face unprecedented challenges in providing adequate support and resources for those diagnosed with Alzheimer's.

This section will explore the staggering statistics, shedding light on the global burden of Alzheimer's. From Asia to the Americas, the prevalence and consequences of the disease will be examined, emphasizing the urgent need for comprehensive research and effective interventions.

Historical Perspectives on Alzheimer's Research

To comprehend the present state of Alzheimer's research, a journey through its historical context becomes imperative. Pioneering efforts to unravel the mysteries of this neurodegenerative disorder have been ongoing for decades. From the early identification of key pathological hallmarks to the evolution of diagnostic criteria, the trajectory of Alzheimer's research provides crucial insights.

The exploration of historical perspectives will involve delving into seminal moments and breakthroughs that have shaped our understanding of the disease. Early misconceptions, scientific advancements, and paradigm shifts will be dissected, creating a narrative that underscores the complexity of Alzheimer's and the relentless pursuit of knowledge by researchers throughout the years.

In retracing the steps of those who laid the foundation for current research endeavors, we gain a deeper appreciation for the challenges faced and the progress made. Historical reflections will set the stage for a comprehensive examination of contemporary investigations into Alzheimer's disease.

As we embark on this intellectual journey, it is with the understanding that the introduction to Alzheimer's goes beyond the scientific realm. It encompasses the collective struggle of individuals and communities affected by the disease, and the dedication of researchers striving to decipher its intricate mechanisms. In the chapters that follow, we will unravel the complexities of neuron loss, RNA dynamics, and novel therapeutic approaches, aiming to contribute to the ongoing narrative of hope and progress in the fight against Alzheimer's.

Chapter 2: Neuron Loss Puzzle

Neuron loss lies at the heart of Alzheimer's disease, contributing to the progressive decline in cognitive functions. To comprehend the complexity of this puzzle, we must embark on a journey into the intricate mechanisms that underlie brain cell death. This chapter delves into the enigma of neuron loss, dissecting its causes and unveiling the role of two key players: amyloid-beta plaques and tau neurofibrillary tangles.

Unraveling the Causes of Brain Cell Death

The quest to unravel the causes of brain cell death in Alzheimer's disease is akin to navigating through a maze of molecular intricacies. Neurons, the building blocks of the brain's communication network, succumb to degeneration, leading to the hallmark cognitive decline. The intricate interplay of genetic, environmental, and age-related factors creates a complex landscape that researchers tirelessly endeavor to decipher.

This section explores the multifaceted nature of neuron loss, delving into the genetic predispositions that may elevate susceptibility. Environmental influences, such as lifestyle and exposure to certain toxins, will be scrutinized for their potential impact on neuronal health. The aging process itself, a fundamental aspect of Alzheimer's, adds another layer to the intricate puzzle, as neurons become more vulnerable over time.

As we journey through the molecular pathways involved in brain cell death, the intricate dance of proteins and the disruption of cellular homeostasis will be unveiled. Understanding the causes of neuron loss is crucial not only for unraveling the mysteries of Alzheimer's but also for identifying potential targets for therapeutic interventions.

Amyloid-Beta Plaques and Tau Neurofibrillary Tangles

Central to the Alzheimer's narrative are the notorious amyloid-beta plaques and tau neurofibrillary tangles, pathological hallmarks that have long captured the attention of researchers. Amyloid-beta, a peptide derived from the amyloid precursor protein, accumulates outside neurons, forming plaques that disrupt communication between cells. Tau, a microtubule-associated protein, undergoes abnormal phosphorylation, leading to the formation of neurofibrillary tangles inside neurons.

This section dissects the intricate relationship between these two players and their role in brain cell death. The amyloid cascade hypothesis, which posits that the accumulation of amyloid-beta initiates a chain reaction leading to tau pathology and neurodegeneration, will be critically examined. Insights from studies on transgenic mouse models and post-mortem human brains will shed light on the dynamic interplay between amyloid-beta and tau.

While amyloid-beta and tau have taken center stage in Alzheimer's research, the relationship between these hallmarks and neuron loss is far from straightforward. This section will explore the nuances of their contributions, addressing the ongoing debate regarding their relative significance and potential as therapeutic targets.

In unraveling the neuron loss puzzle, we navigate through the intricate landscape of molecular events, genetic predispositions, and environmental influences. The journey into the causes of brain cell death is a pivotal step in understanding Alzheimer's disease and holds the promise of uncovering novel avenues for intervention.

As we move forward in this exploration, we transition from the foundational understanding of neuron loss to the next chapter, where the focus shifts to the role of RNA in the intricate dance of cellular processes. The journey into the mysteries of Alzheimer's continues, fueled by a relentless pursuit of knowledge and the hope of finding solutions to one of the most challenging puzzles in neurodegenerative disorders.

Chapter 3: RNA's Dual Role

RNA, the unsung hero of cellular processes, plays a pivotal role in the intricate dance of biological functions. This chapter embarks on a journey into the molecular realm, exploring the significance of Ribonucleic Acids (RNAs) and their dual role in maintaining cellular homeostasis. From their indispensable contributions to protein production to the subtle transition from protective to toxic RNAs with age, the complex landscape of RNA biology unfolds.

Significance of Ribonucleic Acids (RNAs) in Biological Functions

At the heart of cellular orchestration lies the remarkable versatility of RNAs. These molecules, cousins of DNA, are indispensable for the execution of numerous biological functions. While DNA holds the blueprint of life, it is RNA that translates this information into the functional machinery of cells.

This section delves into the diverse roles of RNAs, from the messenger RNA (mRNA) guiding protein synthesis to the ribosomal and transfer RNAs facilitating this intricate process. The regulatory roles of microRNAs and long non-coding RNAs add another layer of complexity, fine-tuning gene expression and influencing cellular fate. Understanding the nuanced interplay of these RNA species is essential for unraveling the mysteries of cellular dynamics.

As we navigate through the significance of RNAs, the focus expands beyond the canonical roles to emerging functions, such as RNA's involvement in cellular signaling and response to stress. The intricate web of RNA-mediated processes sets the stage for exploring how these molecules, once protectors of cellular homeostasis, can undergo a transformative shift, contributing to the complexities of aging and neurodegenerative disorders.

Transition from Protective to Toxic RNAs with Age

Aging, the inevitable journey of biological systems through time, brings about subtle yet profound changes in cellular dynamics. One such transformation involves the transition of RNAs from being protective guardians to potential instigators of cellular havoc. This section unravels the molecular nuances of this transition, shedding light on the role of short strands of RNAs (sRNAs) in the delicate balance between protection and toxicity.

The journey into the aging cellular landscape reveals that as individuals age, the once protective sRNAs can turn into toxic agents. These short RNA strands, which were once instrumental in maintaining cellular health, undergo a shift in their activities. The delicate equilibrium tips toward the toxic side, setting the stage for cellular dysfunction and, in the context of Alzheimer's disease, brain cell death.

The section draws on insights from recent research conducted by Northwestern Medicine, highlighting the groundbreaking discovery that links the activities of sRNAs to Alzheimer's disease. Dr. Marcus Peter and his team at Northwestern University have provided a key piece to the puzzle, uncovering the connection between the imbalance of toxic and protective sRNAs and the development of Alzheimer's.

Understanding this transition is crucial for deciphering the complexities of age-related neurodegenerative diseases. The interplay between protective and toxic sRNAs not only contributes to our understanding of Alzheimer's but also opens new avenues for therapeutic interventions. As we embark on the next phase of research, exploring the specific role of toxic sRNAs in causing cell death, the implications of this discovery extend beyond Alzheimer's to a broader understanding of neurodegenerative diseases and the aging process itself.

In the chapters that follow, we delve into the practical applications of this newfound knowledge. From potential treatments that focus on stabilizing or increasing protective sRNAs to the identification of compounds that could modulate the levels of these RNA species, the journey into the RNA landscape holds promise for innovative approaches to tackling Alzheimer's and related disorders. As we stand at the intersection of molecular biology and neuroscience, the intricate interplay of RNAs takes center stage, offering hope for a deeper understanding and effective interventions in the realm of neurodegeneration.

Chapter 4: sRNAs: The Culprits Revealed

In the intricate tapestry of Alzheimer's disease, short strands of Ribonucleic Acids (sRNAs) emerge as key players, revealing a previously unexplored dimension in the quest to decipher the underlying mechanisms of brain cell death. This chapter embarks on an exploration into the culprits behind neurodegeneration, shedding light on the identification of short strands of toxic RNAs and their profound contribution to brain cell death and DNA damage.

Identifying Short Strands of Toxic RNAs

The enigma of Alzheimer's disease unravels further as researchers uncover the specific culprits that contribute to the devastation of brain cells. In a groundbreaking study by Northwestern Medicine, short strands of toxic RNAs (sRNAs) take center stage. The identification of these molecular instigators provides a critical piece to the puzzle, linking RNA interference to the pathogenesis of Alzheimer's.

This section delves into the methodologies and insights that led to the discovery of toxic sRNAs. Utilizing advanced techniques, researchers at Northwestern University examined the brains of Alzheimer's disease mouse models, young and old mice, as well as neurons from individuals both with and without Alzheimer's. This comprehensive approach allowed them to pinpoint the presence of toxic sRNAs in older patients and those with Alzheimer's, establishing a direct association between these molecular agents and neurodegeneration.

The significance of this identification lies not only in connecting sRNAs to Alzheimer's but also in highlighting their role as potential therapeutic targets. Understanding the characteristics and activities of these toxic RNA strands is a crucial step toward developing interventions that can modulate their impact, offering hope for novel treatments and strategies to halt the progression of Alzheimer's disease.

Contribution to Brain Cell Death and DNA Damage

With the identification of toxic sRNAs comes the realization of their profound contribution to the demise of brain cells and the associated DNA damage. This section dissects the molecular mechanisms through which these short RNA strands instigate cellular dysfunction, ultimately leading to the hallmark of Alzheimer's pathology: brain cell death.

The Northwestern Medicine study illuminates a critical aspect of this contribution – the hindrance of protein production essential for cell survival.

Normally, RNAs play a pivotal role in protein synthesis, ensuring the production of vital components that maintain cellular health. However, the toxic sRNAs identified in Alzheimer's disrupt this process, leading to a cascade of events that culminate in the death of neurons.

As we unravel the intricate dance of cellular processes, it becomes evident that the toxic sRNAs not only contribute to brain cell death but also inflict damage on DNA. The disruption of cellular homeostasis by these molecular culprits sets the stage for a cycle of degeneration, further propagating the progression of Alzheimer's disease.

Understanding the molecular intricacies of how toxic sRNAs induce brain cell death and DNA damage is pivotal for designing targeted therapeutic interventions. This newfound knowledge opens avenues for research aimed at developing compounds or strategies that can either neutralize the impact of toxic sRNAs or enhance the presence of protective sRNAs in the aging brain.

The implications of this discovery extend beyond Alzheimer's disease. By unraveling the specific mechanisms through which toxic sRNAs contribute to neurodegeneration, researchers pave the way for a deeper understanding of similar processes in other neurodegenerative diseases. The identification of common molecular pathways may lead to broad-spectrum therapeutic approaches that address the shared elements of various disorders, bringing us closer to effective treatments for a range of conditions affecting the aging brain.

As we conclude our exploration of sRNAs and their role in Alzheimer's, the journey into the molecular landscape continues. The next chapters will delve into the potential treatments and interventions inspired by these revelations, offering a glimpse into the future of Alzheimer's research and the prospects of innovative therapies that may reshape the landscape of neurodegenerative disease management.

Chapter 5: Shifting Balance in Aging Brain Cells

The delicate balance within aging brain cells holds the key to understanding the progression of Alzheimer's disease. This chapter delves into the intricate dynamics of short strands of Ribonucleic Acids (sRNAs), exploring the transition from protective to toxic states as cells age. By deciphering this shifting equilibrium, we gain profound insights into the mechanisms driving Alzheimer's development.

Understanding the Dynamics of Toxic and Protective sRNAs

Aging, an inevitable biological process, introduces a nuanced interplay between protective and toxic sRNAs in brain cells. This section unravels the dynamics of this delicate equilibrium, shedding light on how the balance tips toward toxicity as cells age. The groundbreaking research from Northwestern Medicine has uncovered the subtle yet impactful changes in the activities of sRNAs within aging brain cells.

As individuals age, the once vigilant protective sRNAs undergo a transformation, shifting their roles toward a toxic trajectory. This transformative process is not a sudden event but a gradual shift, occurring over the course of aging. The mechanisms governing this transition are complex, involving intricate molecular pathways that influence the activities of these short RNA strands.

Researchers are meticulously dissecting the cellular and molecular events that drive this shift, aiming to elucidate the precise triggers and regulators of sRNA dynamics in aging brain cells. By understanding the intricacies of this transition, we move closer to deciphering the underlying causes of Alzheimer's and potentially identifying windows of intervention to disrupt or mitigate the toxic effects of sRNAs.

Implications for Alzheimer's Development

The revelation of the shifting balance in aging brain cells has profound implications for our understanding of Alzheimer's disease development. This section delves into the cascading effects of the altered equilibrium between toxic and protective sRNAs, emphasizing their role as pivotal factors in the onset and progression of Alzheimer's.

The imbalances identified in the Northwestern Medicine study correlate with higher levels of toxic sRNAs in older patients and those diagnosed with Alzheimer's. This correlation suggests a direct link between the shift in sRNA dynamics and the neurodegenerative processes characteristic of Alzheimer's disease. The implications extend beyond mere correlation, hinting at a potential causal relationship that drives the progression of the disease.

The age-related decline in protective sRNAs leaves neurons vulnerable to the damaging effects of toxic sRNAs, contributing to the death of brain cells and the subsequent development of Alzheimer's pathology. Understanding this connection opens new avenues for therapeutic strategies that focus on restoring or enhancing the protective functions of sRNAs in aging brains.

Moreover, the implications of this research transcend Alzheimer's disease, offering insights into the broader landscape of neurodegenerative disorders. The age-dependent shifts in sRNA dynamics may represent a common thread in various conditions affecting the aging brain. Unraveling these shared mechanisms provides a foundation for developing targeted interventions that address the root causes of multiple neurodegenerative diseases.

As we grapple with the complex dynamics of sRNAs in aging brain cells, the research journey leads us toward a deeper understanding of Alzheimer's disease. The intricate dance of protective and toxic sRNAs paints a dynamic portrait of cellular processes, shaping the narrative of neurodegeneration. The next chapters will explore potential therapeutic approaches inspired by these insights, offering hope for innovative interventions that may alter the trajectory of Alzheimer's and related disorders.

Chapter 6: Beyond Traditional Approaches

In the quest for effective treatments for Alzheimer's disease, this chapter ventures beyond traditional approaches that have primarily focused on amyloid plaques and tau tangles. It explores the challenges associated with these conventional methods and introduces the novel concept of RNA interference as a promising therapeutic approach.

Challenges with Amyloid Plaque and Tau-Targeted Treatments

For decades, the lion's share of Alzheimer's research has concentrated on two primary mechanisms: reducing amyloid plaque load and preventing the formation of tau neurofibrillary tangles. While these approaches represent the hallmark features of Alzheimer's diagnosis, the journey toward effective treatments has been fraught with challenges.

This section dissects the difficulties faced in the pursuit of amyloid and tau-targeted treatments. Despite significant investments and efforts, clinical trials centered around reducing amyloid plaque load have yielded limited success. Challenges include the complexity of the disease, late-stage interventions, and the potential multifactorial nature of Alzheimer's pathogenesis. Additionally, the lack of clear causative links between these hallmark features and cognitive decline has prompted a reevaluation of the traditional strategies.

Exploring tau-targeted treatments presents its own set of challenges. Tau pathology, while closely associated with Alzheimer's, introduces a level of intricacy that has proven challenging to address effectively. The complexities of targeting tau, its diverse isoforms, and its role in normal cellular functions pose significant hurdles for therapeutic development.

Acknowledging these challenges opens the door to alternative approaches, emphasizing the need for innovative strategies that can potentially address the root causes of Alzheimer's disease.

Exploring RNA Interference as a Novel Therapeutic Approach

Amidst the challenges posed by traditional approaches, a novel therapeutic concept emerges: RNA interference (RNAi). This section introduces the exploration of RNAi as a groundbreaking method to tackle Alzheimer's disease, inspired by recent revelations about the role of short RNA strands (sRNAs) in neurodegeneration.

The Northwestern Medicine study, uncovering the connection between toxic sRNAs and brain cell death, has paved the way for considering RNAi as a potential game-changer. RNAi allows for the selective silencing or modulation of specific RNA sequences, offering a targeted and precision-oriented approach to intervene in the cellular processes driving Alzheimer's pathology.

By honing in on the molecular culprits, specifically toxic sRNAs identified in the aging brain, RNAi presents an opportunity to disrupt the cascade of events leading to neuron loss. The feasibility of manipulating RNA dynamics offers a novel avenue for therapeutic development that transcends the limitations of traditional approaches.

The potential of RNA interference extends beyond Alzheimer's disease. As researchers delve deeper into the molecular landscape of sRNAs, the insights gained may have broader applications in understanding and treating various neurodegenerative disorders. RNAi-based therapies could offer a versatile platform for addressing shared molecular mechanisms across different conditions affecting the aging brain.

While RNA interference introduces a promising frontier in Alzheimer's research, challenges lie ahead. Refining the specificity and delivery mechanisms of RNAi therapies, ensuring their safety and efficacy, and navigating the complexities of translating these approaches from bench to bedside are critical considerations. However, the potential benefits of a targeted, precision-oriented intervention make RNA interference an exciting avenue for further exploration and development.

As we venture beyond traditional approaches, the landscape of Alzheimer's research evolves. The challenges with amyloid and tau-centric strategies prompt a paradigm shift toward innovative methods inspired by the molecular revelations of sRNAs. The next chapters will explore the practical implications and potential applications of RNA interference, offering a glimpse into the future of Alzheimer's therapeutics and the transformative possibilities that may reshape the landscape of neurodegenerative disease management.

Chapter 7: New Horizons in Alzheimer's Treatment

As we stand at the cusp of groundbreaking discoveries, this chapter delves into the new horizons in Alzheimer's treatment. Exploring the potential of stabilizing or increasing protective short strands of Ribonucleic Acids (sRNAs), it charts alternative strategies for halting or delaying the relentless progression of Alzheimer's disease. This represents a paradigm shift in therapeutic perspectives, inspired by recent insights into the delicate balance of sRNAs and their impact on neurodegeneration.

Potential of Stabilizing or Increasing Protective sRNAs

The newfound understanding of the critical role played by protective sRNAs in maintaining cellular health opens the door to innovative therapeutic strategies. This section navigates through the potential of stabilizing or increasing protective sRNAs as a novel approach to counteract Alzheimer's disease.

The delicate equilibrium between toxic and protective sRNAs within aging brain cells has emerged as a key determinant in the development of Alzheimer's. By focusing on enhancing the levels or stabilizing the activities of protective sRNAs, researchers aim to tip the balance back toward cellular health. This represents a departure from traditional approaches that predominantly targeted amyloid plaques and tau tangles.

The feasibility of such an approach relies on a deeper understanding of the regulatory mechanisms governing protective sRNAs. Researchers are now exploring ways to modulate these molecules, investigating whether external interventions can effectively enhance their protective functions. The potential impact of this strategy extends not only to Alzheimer's but also to a broader spectrum of neurodegenerative diseases, offering a targeted and nuanced approach to intervention.

As we envision the potential of stabilizing or increasing protective sRNAs, the practical implications include the development of therapeutics that could potentially slow down or even reverse the neurodegenerative processes observed in Alzheimer's. The journey into this uncharted territory opens up new vistas for treatment modalities that aim to address the root causes of the disease, marking a paradigm shift in Alzheimer's therapeutics.

Alternative Strategies for Halting or Delaying Alzheimer's

Traditional treatment approaches for Alzheimer's, primarily centered around amyloid and tau-targeted strategies, have faced significant challenges. In light of these difficulties, this section explores alternative strategies for halting or delaying the progression of Alzheimer's disease. Inspired by the recent revelations about sRNAs, these alternative approaches seek to break new ground in the pursuit of effective interventions.

The shift in focus toward sRNAs introduces a range of alternative strategies that challenge the conventional understanding of Alzheimer's pathology. By recognizing the multifaceted nature of the disease, researchers are exploring diversified approaches that go beyond targeting singular hallmark features. This includes interventions aimed at modulating the balance of toxic and protective sRNAs, as well as strategies inspired by RNA interference.

One alternative avenue involves the identification of small molecules or compounds that can influence sRNA dynamics in a beneficial way. Researchers are actively searching for substances that can enhance protective sRNA levels or inhibit the activities of toxic counterparts. This approach aligns with the growing emphasis on precision medicine, tailoring interventions to the specific molecular imbalances observed in individuals with Alzheimer's.

Additionally, the exploration of gene therapies and innovative delivery methods holds promise in the realm of alternative strategies. The goal is to develop interventions that can be administered early in the disease process, potentially even before clinical symptoms manifest. This proactive approach aims to halt or slow down the neurodegenerative cascade, marking a departure from reactive treatments focused on symptomatic relief.

The implications of these alternative strategies are transformative, offering hope for more effective and personalized treatments for Alzheimer's disease. As the research community continues to unravel the complexities of sRNAs and their role in neurodegeneration, the landscape of Alzheimer's treatment undergoes a profound shift toward precision-oriented and targeted interventions.

In the chapters that follow, we will explore the practical applications and ongoing research endeavors inspired by these new horizons. From the development of therapeutics that harness the potential of protective sRNAs to the exploration of alternative strategies that challenge traditional norms, the future of Alzheimer's treatment is characterized by innovation and a deeper understanding of the molecular intricacies driving neurodegeneration.

Chapter 8: Widening Perspectives

This chapter expands the lens through which we view Alzheimer's disease, exploring its implications beyond the immediate focus on sRNAs and neurodegeneration. By examining the potential impact on treating other neurodegenerative diseases and unraveling the mysteries surrounding decades of symptom-free life followed by the onset of neurodegeneration, we enter a realm that widens our perspectives on the intricate landscape of age-related cognitive decline.

Implications for Treating Other Neurodegenerative Diseases

The journey into understanding the role of sRNAs in Alzheimer's disease unveils broader implications for treating a spectrum of neurodegenerative diseases. This section delves into how the insights gained from the study of sRNAs can be translated into potential therapeutic approaches for conditions beyond Alzheimer's.

The shared molecular pathways and common mechanisms observed in various neurodegenerative diseases create a foundation for exploring interventions that go beyond the boundaries of specific conditions. The identification of protective and toxic sRNAs, their imbalances, and their role in cellular health may serve as a unifying theme in the search for treatments targeting age-related cognitive decline.

As researchers uncover the intricacies of sRNAs, the hope is that these findings can be translated into broader therapeutic strategies applicable to conditions such as Parkinson's disease, Huntington's disease, and other forms of dementia. By addressing shared molecular mechanisms, researchers aim to develop interventions that have the potential to impact a range of neurodegenerative disorders, marking a significant step toward comprehensive and versatile treatments.

Understanding the implications for treating other neurodegenerative diseases not only enhances the breadth of therapeutic applications but also fosters a collaborative and interdisciplinary approach to research. As the boundaries between different conditions blur, the collective effort to decipher the mysteries of sRNAs may pave the way for transformative treatments that transcend individual diseases.

Decades of Symptom-Free Life and the Onset of Neurodegeneration

One of the most intriguing aspects of neurodegenerative diseases, including Alzheimer's, is the phenomenon of decades of symptom-free life followed by the gradual onset of cognitive decline. This section explores the mysteries surrounding this temporal gap and how the insights into sRNAs may offer clues to unravel this enigma.

The typical trajectory of neurodegenerative diseases often involves a prolonged period during which individuals appear asymptomatic. This "preclinical" phase poses a challenge for early diagnosis and intervention. The Northwestern Medicine study's findings on the shifting balance of sRNAs and the role they play in brain cell death raise questions about what triggers the transition from a seemingly healthy state to neurodegeneration.

Researchers are now investigating whether the age-related decline in protective sRNAs and the concurrent rise in toxic counterparts contribute to this asymptomatic phase. The subtle molecular changes occurring during these decades of apparent health may hold the key to understanding the early stages of neurodegenerative diseases.

By exploring the intricate dance of sRNAs in this preclinical phase, researchers aim to identify potential biomarkers or early indicators that can signal the onset of neurodegeneration long before clinical symptoms emerge. This proactive approach could revolutionize early diagnosis and intervention strategies, offering the possibility of treatments that can slow down or halt the progression of neurodegenerative diseases during their earliest stages.

The implications of unraveling the mysteries surrounding decades of symptom-free life extend beyond Alzheimer's to the broader landscape of aging and cognitive health. By connecting the dots between sRNAs, the preclinical phase, and the onset of neurodegeneration, researchers aim to redefine our understanding of the aging process and open avenues for interventions that can preserve cognitive function throughout the lifespan.

As we widen our perspectives, the focus on sRNAs transcends individual diseases and timelines. The interconnectedness of these insights not only enhances our understanding of neurodegenerative disorders but also fuels a collective endeavor to transform the landscape of cognitive health. The chapters that follow will delve into the practical applications of these widened perspectives, exploring the potential for innovative treatments and strategies that may reshape the narrative of aging and neurodegeneration.

Chapter 9: Unraveling the Role of Toxic sRNAs

In the intricate landscape of Alzheimer's disease, short strands of Ribonucleic Acids (sRNAs) emerge as pivotal players, especially the toxic variants. This chapter delves into the nuanced exploration of the specific contributions of toxic sRNAs, guiding us through the next steps in research. As we venture into the realms of animal models and the brains of Alzheimer's patients, we seek to unravel the intricacies of toxic sRNA activities that underlie the neurodegenerative processes in this devastating condition.

Next Steps in Research: Animal Models and Alzheimer's Patient Brains

The journey to understand the role of toxic sRNAs necessitates a comprehensive approach, embracing insights from both controlled experimental settings and the complex reality of human brains affected by Alzheimer's. This section intricately explores the next steps in research, highlighting the significance of studying animal models and delving into the brains of individuals diagnosed with Alzheimer's.

Animal models stand as indispensable tools in neuroscientific exploration, offering controlled environments where researchers can manipulate variables to understand intricate biological processes. In the realm of toxic sRNAs, genetically modified mice and other model organisms provide invaluable insights. Researchers can experimentally alter sRNA levels, observe resultant effects on brain cells, and unravel the specific mechanisms through which toxic sRNAs contribute to neurodegeneration.

However, the translation of findings from animal models to the complex human condition requires a parallel investigation in post-mortem brains from individuals diagnosed with Alzheimer's. This approach enables researchers to validate insights gleaned from animal studies and appreciate the nuances of toxic sRNA activities within the context of the disease's heterogeneity.

The marriage of animal model studies with analyses of human brain tissue creates a synergistic research approach. This combination bridges the gap between controlled experiments and the intricate reality of Alzheimer's pathology. It allows for a more nuanced understanding of how toxic sRNAs influence neurodegeneration, considering the subtleties that arise in the human brain's complex and diverse landscape.

As researchers unravel the role of toxic sRNAs in this integrated approach, they move closer to comprehending the molecular intricacies underpinning Alzheimer's disease. The insights gained from studying both animal models and human brains provide a more holistic understanding, essential for the development of targeted and effective therapeutic strategies.

Identifying Compounds to Modulate sRNA Levels

In the quest to harness the potential of sRNAs for therapeutic interventions, identifying compounds capable of modulating their levels emerges as a pivotal endeavor. This section embarks on the exploration of ongoing efforts to pinpoint substances that can selectively alter the balance of toxic and protective sRNAs. The goal is to pave the way for innovative therapeutic strategies that may revolutionize the landscape of Alzheimer's disease treatment.

The identification of compounds capable of modulating sRNA levels represents a critical juncture in Alzheimer's research. The delicate equilibrium between toxic and protective sRNAs within aging brain cells is poised for intervention. Researchers are diligently screening libraries of small molecules and exploring natural compounds, aiming to identify substances that can either enhance protective sRNAs or inhibit the activities of their toxic counterparts.

This targeted approach holds significant promise, seeking to restore the delicate balance within aging brain cells and counteract the neurodegenerative processes associated with Alzheimer's disease. The screening process involves a meticulous evaluation of numerous compounds in cellular and animal models, assessing their efficacy, safety, and specificity in modulating sRNA dynamics.

The quest to identify compounds to modulate sRNA levels is not only about addressing Alzheimer's but also extends to the broader landscape of neurodegenerative diseases. The exploration of these compounds opens possibilities for developing broad-spectrum treatments that target shared molecular mechanisms across various conditions affecting the aging brain.

The screening process involves the assessment of safety and efficacy, ensuring that any identified compounds have the potential for translational applications. The ultimate goal is to translate these findings into innovative therapeutic strategies, moving beyond conventional approaches that primarily target symptoms.

As we delve into the practical applications of these findings, the next chapters will explore the potential translation of research discoveries into clinical practice. From the development of targeted therapeutics to the intricacies of clinical trials, the exploration of toxic sRNAs takes us one step closer to innovative solutions for Alzheimer's and related neurodegenerative conditions.

Chapter 10: Conclusion

In this concluding chapter, we reflect on the intricate journey through the landscape of Alzheimer's disease, exploring the role of short strands of Ribonucleic Acids (sRNAs) and their potential impact on future treatments. The road traversed through unraveling the complexities of toxic sRNAs has led to profound insights, and as we conclude, we examine the road ahead in Alzheimer's research. We also peer into the hopeful prospects that these revelations hold for future treatments, marking a transformative era in the pursuit of effective interventions for this prevalent and devastating neurodegenerative condition.

The Road Ahead in Alzheimer's Research

As we stand at the culmination of this exploration, the road ahead in Alzheimer's research stretches before us, illuminated by the discoveries made in the realm of sRNAs. The journey has been one of intricate unraveling, bringing to light the molecular intricacies that underlie the devastating progression of Alzheimer's disease.

The road ahead is paved with promise and challenges alike. The identification of toxic sRNAs and their role in brain cell death opens new vistas for research avenues. The integration of findings from animal models and studies on Alzheimer's patient brains sets the stage for a more comprehensive understanding of the disease's nuances. However, with this newfound knowledge comes the responsibility to translate it into practical applications that can tangibly impact the lives of those affected by Alzheimer's.

One key aspect of the road ahead involves further elucidating the precise mechanisms through which toxic sRNAs contribute to neurodegeneration. Researchers will delve deeper into the molecular dance of these short RNA strands, seeking to uncover additional factors and interactions that influence their activities. Understanding these intricate details is crucial for designing targeted interventions that can disrupt the cascade of events leading to brain cell death.

Moreover, the road ahead necessitates a continued commitment to translational research. Bridging the gap between laboratory discoveries and clinical applications requires a concerted effort to develop therapies inspired by the insights gained from sRNA studies. Clinical trials will play a pivotal role in assessing the safety and efficacy of potential treatments, offering a bridge between the laboratory and the patient's bedside.

Collaboration across disciplines and research institutions will be paramount in navigating the complexities of Alzheimer's disease. The integration of expertise from molecular biology, neuroscience, clinical medicine, and other relevant fields will foster a holistic approach to understanding and treating this multifaceted condition. The road ahead is not solitary but a collective endeavor that unites researchers, clinicians, and advocates in the common pursuit of advancing Alzheimer's research.

Hopeful Prospects for Future Treatments

Amidst the challenges, the revelations surrounding toxic sRNAs bring forth hopeful prospects for the future of Alzheimer's treatments. This section explores the transformative potential of these insights, offering a glimpse into the possibilities that may reshape the landscape of neurodegenerative disease management.

The identification of toxic sRNAs has introduced a paradigm shift in our understanding of Alzheimer's pathology. The hope lies in the potential to develop targeted therapeutic interventions that address the root causes of the disease. By modulating sRNA levels, researchers envision a future where the delicate balance within aging brain cells can be restored, halting or delaying the neurodegenerative processes that lead to cognitive decline.

One of the hopeful prospects lies in the development of precision-oriented treatments inspired by the nuances of sRNA dynamics. Researchers aim to identify compounds that can selectively enhance protective sRNAs or inhibit the activities of toxic counterparts. This targeted approach holds the promise of personalized interventions tailored to the specific molecular imbalances observed in individuals with Alzheimer's.

Furthermore, the newfound understanding of toxic sRNAs opens avenues for innovative therapeutic strategies, such as RNA interference. The ability to selectively silence or modulate specific RNA sequences provides a powerful tool for intervening in the molecular processes driving Alzheimer's pathology. As researchers continue to refine these approaches, the prospect of RNA-based therapeutics emerges as a transformative possibility for the future.

Hope also lies in the potential application of these insights to other neurodegenerative diseases. The shared molecular mechanisms observed in various conditions affecting the aging brain suggest that interventions targeting toxic sRNAs may have broader implications. This interconnected perspective offers a ray of optimism for developing treatments that can address common elements across different neurodegenerative disorders.

Clinical trials will play a pivotal role in translating these hopeful prospects into tangible treatments. The rigorous evaluation of safety and efficacy in human subjects is essential for bringing potential therapies from the laboratory bench to the patient's bedside. The collaborative efforts of researchers, clinicians, and pharmaceutical partners will be instrumental in advancing these treatments through the complex phases of clinical development.

The integration of sRNA insights into the broader landscape of Alzheimer's research also holds potential for early diagnosis and prevention. If the age-related decline in protective sRNAs is identified as an early indicator of neurodegeneration, it could revolutionize the approach to detecting and intervening in Alzheimer's disease during its preclinical stages.

In conclusion, the journey through the intricate world of sRNAs in Alzheimer's disease opens a chapter of hope and possibility. The road ahead in Alzheimer's research is characterized by ongoing discovery, collaboration, and the pursuit of innovative treatments. The hopeful prospects for future interventions inspired by toxic sRNA insights signify a transformative era in the quest to conquer Alzheimer's and offer renewed hope for individuals and families affected by this challenging condition.